T0065187

HARMONY IN HORMONES:

A COMPREHENSIVE GUIDE TO MENOPAUSE TREATMENT

HARMONY IN HORMONES:

A COMPREHENSIVE GUIDE TO MENOPAUSE TREATMENT

Empowering Women Through Hormone Replacement Therapy

DEREK LAMBERT, NP

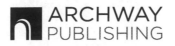

ARCHWAY PUBLISHING

Archway Publishing books may be ordered through booksellers or by contacting:

Archway Publishing
1663 Liberty Drive
Bloomington, IN 47403
www.archwaypublishing.com
844-669-3957

ISBN: 978-1-6657-5515-3 (sc)
ISBN: 978-1-6657-5514-6 (e)

Library of Congress Control Number: 2024900291

Print information available on the last page.

Archway Publishing rev. date: 01/10/2024

Legal & Disclaimer

The information contained in this book and its contents is not designed to replace or take the place of any form of medical or professional advice; and is not meant to replace the need for independent medical, financial, legal or other professional advice or services, as may be required. The content and information in this book has been provided for educational and entertainment purposes only.

The content and information contained in this book has been compiled from sources deemed reliable, and it is accurate to the best of the Author's knowledge, information and belief. However, the Author cannot guarantee its accuracy and validity and cannot be held liable for any errors and/or omissions. Further, changes are periodically made to this book as and when needed. Where appropriate and/or necessary, you must consult a professional (including but not limited to your doctor, attorney, financial advisor or such other professional advisor) before using any of the suggested remedies, techniques, or information in this book.

Upon using the contents and information contained in this book, you agree to hold harmless the Author from and against any damages, costs, and expenses, including any legal fees potentially resulting from the application of any of the information provided by this book. This disclaimer applies to any loss, damages or injury caused by the use and application, whether directly or indirectly, of any advice or information presented, whether for breach of contract, tort, negligence, personal injury, criminal intent, or under any other cause of action.

You agree to accept all risks of using the information presented inside this book.

You agree that by continuing to read this book, where appropriate and/or necessary, you shall consult a professional (including but not limited to your doctor, attorney, or financial advisor or such other advisor as needed) before using any of the suggested remedies, techniques, or information in this book.

Contents

Introduction

"Harmony in Hormones: Empowering Women Through Hormone Replacement Therapy" is a comprehensive guide that takes you on an enlightening journey through the complexities of menopause treatment and the transformative potential of Hormone Replacement Therapy (HRT). It begins by exploring menopause, a natural and inevitable phase in a woman's life that represents a significant shift in hormonal balance. In this section, we'll provide a concise yet thorough overview of menopause, unraveling the biological intricacies and shedding light on the diverse symptoms that accompany this transformative journey. Understanding the challenges and changes of menopause sets the stage for the empowering solutions found in Hormone Replacement Therapy.

HRT plays a pivotal role in restoring hormonal balance and emerges as a beacon of hope and empowerment in the menopausal landscape. This segment will delve into the transformative role of HRT, exploring its historical context, evolution, and the benefits it offers in alleviating symptoms and enhancing the overall quality of life for women navigating the complexities of menopause.

Allow me to introduce myself as we delve into the unfolding narrative. I am a nurse practitioner who holds a strong dedication to women's health, specializing specifically in menopause treatment. Through my clinic, I have had the privilege of witnessing the profound impact that personalized care and hormone replacement therapy (HRT) have had on the lives of numerous women. Utilizing my extensive experience, I am fully committed to providing a comprehensive and empathetic approach to menopause care.

This guide goes beyond being a mere collection of facts; it serves as a testament to the tangible success stories that have emerged from the genuine connection between healthcare professionals and the women we are privileged to serve. I invite you to embark on this journey with me, exploring the realm of "Harmony in Hormones," where knowledge empowers and the experience acts as a bridge to a vibrant and fulfilling menopausal life.

Chapter 1

Initiating the Onset of Menopause

M enopause is characterized by the absence of menstrual periods for a period of 12 months. The time before menopause when women have changes in their periods, hot flashes, and other symptoms is called perimenopause. Most women start going through menopause between the ages of 45 and 55. The transition generally takes around seven years but can last up to 14 years depending on the person's smoking habits, the age it starts, ethnicity, and race. In perimenopause, the body produces less estrogen and progesterone, two hormones produced by the ovaries.

As a result of the ovaries releasing fewer reproductive hormones, especially estrogen and progesterone, there is a transitional period that often occurs in the late 40s to early 50s. Recognizing that menopause is a journey with profound implications on a woman's physical, emotional, and mental health rather than merely the end of her menstrual cycle is essential.

Common Menopausal Symptoms and How They Affect Women's Lives

Menopause is a natural and inevitable phase in a woman's life that marks the end of her reproductive years. This transformative journey is characterized by a variety of physical and emotional symptoms that can significantly impact different aspects of a woman's life. It is crucial to understand and address these symptoms to provide effective care and support during this transitional period.

Physical Symptoms:

I.   **Hot Flashes and Night Sweats:** Sudden, intense feelings of heat, often accompanied by sweating, especially during the night. Disrupted sleep patterns, fatigue, and discomfort can affect daily activities, leading to irritability and reduced overall well-being.

II. **Vaginal Dryness:** Reduced lubrication in the vaginal area, leading to discomfort, itching, and pain during intercourse. Sexual intimacy may become challenging, impacting relationships and contributing to emotional distress.

III. **Bladder control:** Controlling when you pee. Incontinence is the inability to maintain control over your bladder. You may experience a sudden urge to urinate or have urine leakage during physical activity, sneezing, or laughing. The first course of action for dealing with incontinence is to consult with a healthcare professional. Middle-aged individuals can also experience bladder infections.

IV. **Changes in Sleep Patterns:** Insomnia, difficulty falling or staying asleep, and increased nighttime awakenings. Fatigue, irritability, and decreased cognitive function can affect work performance and overall quality of life.

V.   **Joint Pain and Muscle Aches:** Increased susceptibility to joint pain and muscle stiffness. Reduced physical activity, potential weight gain, and a decrease in overall mobility and flexibility.

VI. **Changes in Skin Elasticity:** Loss of collagen and changes in skin texture, leading to dryness and increased wrinkles.

Affecting self-esteem and body image, contributing to emotional challenges during this transitional phase.

VII. **Mood Changes:** You might feel more easily annoyed or upset during menopause. It remains a mystery to researchers why this occurs, your mood may be affected by feeling stressed, changes in your family, such as children aging or parents getting older, previous experience with depression, or fatigue. Have a conversation with your primary care provider, physician, or counselor regarding your current situation. There are ways to help with the problem.

VIII. **Body Changes:** It may appear like your physique is different. It's possible for your waist to grow. It's possible to acquire fat and lose muscle. You might have thinner skin. In addition to stiffness and aches in your joints and muscles, you may experience memory issues. Scholars are investigating these alterations and their correlation with aging and hormones.

Emotional and Psychological Symptoms:

I. **Mood Swings and Irritability:** Unpredictable mood fluctuations, ranging from sadness to irritability.
   • **Impact:** Strained relationships, increased stress, and challenges in interpersonal interactions.

II. **Anxiety and Depression:** Heightened feelings of anxiety and, in some cases, clinical depression.
   • **Impact:** Impaired mental well-being.

III. **Memory and Concentration Issues:** Cognitive changes, such as forgetfulness and difficulty concentrating.
   • **Impact:** Challenges in work-related tasks and daily responsibilities, leading to frustration and decreased self-confidence.

IV. **Decreased Libido:** Reduced interest or desire for sexual activity.
  - **Impact:** Strain on intimate relationships, potential emotional distress, and changes in self-perception.

The Importance of Seeking Treatment for Menopause

Menopause, a natural and unavoidable stage in a woman's life, can have a significant impact on physical health, emotional well-being, and overall quality of life due to the associated symptoms. Seeking treatment during this phase is crucial as it empowers women to embrace menopause with vitality and resilience. Here are several key reasons why seeking treatment is of the utmost importance:

1. **Relieving Menopausal Symptoms:**
   a) **Physical Comfort:** Treatment options, including Hormone Replacement Therapy (HRT), effectively alleviate common physical symptoms like hot flashes, night sweats, vaginal dryness, and joint pain. This promotes physical comfort and improves sleep quality.
   b) **Emotional Well-being:** Managing emotional symptoms such as mood swings, anxiety, and depression contributes to enhanced emotional well-being, fostering a positive mindset during this transitional phase.

2. **Enhancing Quality of Life:**
   a) **Improved Sleep:** Addressing sleep disturbances through treatment positively impacts energy levels, cognitive function, and overall quality of life.
   b) **Sexual Health:** Treating symptoms like vaginal dryness and decreased libido can improve sexual health, fostering intimate relationships and overall life satisfaction.

3. **Preventing Long-term Health Complications:**
   a) **Bone Health:** Menopausal hormonal changes can affect bone density. Treatment, including adequate calcium and vitamin D supplementation, can help maintain strong and healthy bones, reducing the risk of osteoporosis.
   b) **Cardiovascular Health:** Estrogen, a key hormone affected by menopause, plays a role in cardiovascular health. Treatment strategies can potentially mitigate cardiovascular risks associated with hormonal changes.

4. **Supporting Mental Well-being:** Addressing cognitive symptoms such as memory issues and difficulty concentrating supports mental clarity and cognitive function, contributing to a sense of control and confidence.

Managing emotional symptoms is crucial for maintaining emotional resilience during menopause. This helps prevent the negative impact of anxiety and depression on mental well-being, enabling women to navigate the challenges of this life phase with resilience. Seeking treatment for menopause is an opportunity for individualized and holistic care. Personalized treatment plans, including Hormone Replacement Therapy, consider specific symptoms and health needs. A holistic approach to treatment addresses the physical, emotional, and psychological aspects of a woman's well-being, promoting a balanced and comprehensive care model.

Informed decision-making and active participation in healthcare decisions empower women to make choices aligned with their values, preferences, and health goals. By addressing menopausal symptoms through treatment, women can improve their quality of life, maintain social connections, and continue to lead fulfilling lives. Ultimately, seeking menopause treatment is a proactive step towards embracing this life phase with vitality, well-being, and empowerment.

Chapter 2

Enhancing Menopausal Health with Hormone Replacement Therapy (HRT)

M enopause is a natural phase in a woman's life that can bring about a range of physical and emotional changes due to hormonal fluctuations. Hormone Replacement Therapy (HRT) is a transformative intervention that aims to alleviate symptoms, enhance quality of life, and empower women to navigate this life stage with resilience and vitality.

Understanding Hormone Replacement Therapy:

Principles of HRT:

HRT involves supplementing hormones, such as estrogen, progesterone, and sometimes testosterone, to address imbalances that occur during menopause. The primary goal is to mitigate symptoms arising from hormonal decline, offering relief from hot flashes, night sweats, mood swings, and other menopausal challenges.

Forms of HRT Administration:

HRT can be administered in various forms, including pills, patches, creams, gels, or pellets implanted under the skin. The choice of administration depends on individual preferences, medical history, and the specific hormonal needs of each woman.

There have been concerns regarding the potential link between HRT and an increased risk of breast cancer. It is crucial to understand the nuances of this association, including factors such as the specific type of HRT used and the duration of its use. Regular breast cancer screening and ongoing discussions with healthcare providers are essential in addressing these concerns.

The timing of initiating HRT in relation to the onset of menopause is an important consideration. Starting HRT closer to the onset of menopause may have different risks and benefits compared to starting it later. It is necessary to carefully evaluate the individual's circumstances and make an informed decision based on their specific needs and medical history.

Hormone Replacement Therapy (HRT) Success Stories from Real Patients' Experiences

Perhaps the most moving and authentic testimonies and real-life success stories highlight the revolutionary effects of Hormone Replacement Therapy (HRT) on women's lives. These accounts highlight the personal empowerment and enhanced well-being that women receiving HRT experience in addition to offering a glimpse into the treatment's concrete advantages.

1. **Rediscovering Vitality: Anna's Story:**

52-year-old Anna was having a hard time with intense hot flashes and sleep issues, which were affecting her relationships and career.

Her hot flashes significantly decreased after she started taking HRT, which let her get a good night's sleep again. Anna discovered that she was taking on life's obstacles with fresh vigor, both in her personal and professional life.

2. Improving Mental Health: Testimonial from Sarah:

During her menopause transition, 48-year-old Sarah experienced mood swings and increased anxiety. Her moods were controlled and she felt emotionally balanced thanks to HRT. "HRT helped me feel like myself again, I could interact with life in a more optimistic attitude when the emotional roller coaster subsided. The difference was enormous."

3. Strengthening Close Bonds: Emily's Path:

When it came to her personal relationships, 58 year-old Emily suffered from diminished libido and vaginal dryness. She added hormone replacement therapy (HRT) to her treatment regimen under the advice of her physician. As Emily says, "HRT helped me feel closer and more intimate with my partner again. Sensation of connection and vibrancy is more important than just bodily ease."

4. Regaining Mental Clarity: Rebecca's Story

Rebecca, 55, observed changes in her cognitive abilities, such as trouble focusing and forgetfulness. Her memory and mental clarity improved with HRT customized to meet her individual needs. "It seems like a fog lifting," she says. "I feel more in charge and concentrated. My cognitive health has changed dramatically as a result of HRT."

5. **Handling Somatic Symptoms: Grace's Account:**

Grace, 49, struggled with sleep disturbances and joint pain. Not only did HRT help with these bodily problems, but it also improved her health in general. "I wake up feeling rejuvenated, and I can move without discomfort," she says, "I can now live an active lifestyle again thanks to HRT."

6. **A feeling of empowerment: Linda's path to empowerment:**

53-year-old Linda saw her menopause experience as a chance for personal development. Her comprehensive care plan included HRT, which served as an empowerment tool. She says, "I felt empowered to know my alternatives and to actively participate in my healthcare decisions. HRT turned out to be a wise decision that gave me the confidence to enjoy this stage of life."

These testimonies and real-life success stories highlight the various ways that hormone replacement therapy has improved the lives of women. HRT shows itself to be a useful and empowering tool in negotiating the intricacies of menopause, with benefits ranging from enhanced relationships and a revitalized sense of vigor to physical comfort and mental stability. The choice to pursue HRT should be decided in cooperation with a healthcare provider based on specific health needs and concerns, as individual experiences with the medication can differ.

When used intelligently and under the supervision of medical professionals, hormone replacement therapy (HRT) provides a personalized, all-encompassing approach to addressing the issues associated with menopause.

The Role of Estrogen, Progesterone, and Testosterone In Menopause

In this section, we will explore the intricate realm of hormones, specifically estrogen, progesterone, and testosterone, which are vital components in the symphony of the female body. Understanding the distinct roles that each hormone plays is crucial in comprehending the subtle changes that occur during menopause and the transformative effects of Hormone Replacement Therapy (HRT).

Estrogen: The Mastermind of Femininity

Estrogen is a vital hormone that plays a significant role in the reproductive systems of both males and females. In females, it not only contributes to reproductive and breast health but also has an impact on cognitive health, bone health, cardiovascular function, and various other essential bodily processes. While estrogen is involved in numerous functions, it is commonly recognized for its partnership with progesterone in maintaining female sexual and reproductive health.

Estrogen is produced by the ovaries, adrenal glands, and fat tissues. Although both males and females have this hormone, females naturally produce higher levels of estrogen. This section delves deeper into the intricacies of estrogen, exploring its mechanisms, the consequences of fluctuating levels, and its medical applications.

Types of Estrogen

There are several types of estrogen:

i. **Estrone:** This type of estrogen is prevalent in the body after menopause. It is a lesser form of estrogen that the body can convert to other forms of estrogen as needed.

ii. **Estradiol:** Estradiol is produced by both males and females and is the most frequent form of estrogen in females during their reproductive years. Too much estradiol can cause acne, lack of sex drive, osteoporosis, and depression. Extremely high levels may raise the risk of uterine and breast cancer. Low levels, on the other hand, can cause weight gain and cardiovascular disease.

iii. **Estriol:** Estriol levels rise during pregnancy as the uterus grows and the body prepares for birth. Estriol levels are highest right before delivery.

Function of Estrogen

Estrogen plays a crucial role in the functioning of various organs:

I. **Uterus:** Estrogen enhances and sustains the mucous membrane lining the uterus. Additionally, it regulates the flow and thickness of uterine mucus secretions.

II. **Ovaries:** Estrogen aids in the stimulation of egg follicle growth.

III. **Breasts:** Estrogen is involved in the development of breast tissue. Furthermore, this hormone assists in ceasing milk production after weaning.

IV. **Vagina:** Within the vagina, estrogen is responsible for preserving the thickness of the vaginal wall and promoting lubrication.

The Role of Estrogen in the Female Body:

i. **Reproductive System:** Estrogen plays a pivotal role in the menstrual cycle by regulating the development of the uterine lining and preparing the body for potential pregnancy.

ii. **Bone Health:** It supports bone density, reducing the risk of osteoporosis. Estrogen aids in maintaining adequate levels of calcium and phosphorus, which are essential for strong bones.

iii. **Cardiovascular Health:** Estrogen has a protective effect on the cardiovascular system, influencing cholesterol levels and promoting optimal blood vessel function.

iv. **Skin and Hair:** It contributes to maintaining skin elasticity and hydration, resulting in a youthful complexion. Estrogen also influences hair growth and texture.

Impact of Estrogen Decline in Menopause:

- **Hot Flashes and Night Sweats:** The decline of estrogen is closely associated with the well-known hot flashes and night sweats, which disrupt the body's temperature regulation.

- **Vaginal Dryness:** Estrogen's role in maintaining vaginal lubrication diminishes, leading to discomfort and potential challenges in sexual intimacy.

- **Bone Loss:** Decreased estrogen levels contribute to a decline in bone density, increasing the risk of fractures and osteoporosis.

An excess or deficiency of estrogen can result in a range of symptoms, including irregular or absent periods, heavy or light bleeding during menstruation, intensified premenstrual or menopausal symptoms, hot flashes, night sweats, noncancerous growths in the uterus and breast, mood changes, sleeping difficulties, weight gain in the hips, thighs, and waist, low libido, vaginal dryness and atrophy, fatigue, mood swings, feelings of depression and anxiety, and dry skin. Many of these symptoms are typical during menopause.

Below are some frequently asked questions about estrogen:

1. What are the effects of estrogen on the body?

Estrogen plays a role in various bodily functions, including:

- Stimulating the growth of egg follicles
- Maintaining vaginal lubrication and the thickness of the vaginal wall
- Sustaining the mucous membrane in the uterus
- Contributing to the development of breast tissue

2. **What are the effects of high estrogen levels in females?**

Elevated levels of estradiol, a type of estrogen, can lead to the following:

- Acne
- Decreased sex drive
- Depression
- Increased risk of uterine and breast cancer

3. **What happens if someone has low estrogen?**

Insufficient levels of estradiol may contribute to weight gain and cardiovascular disease. An estrogen imbalance can also result in symptoms such as:

- Changes in menstruation
- Hot flashes
- Mood changes
- Decreased sex drive
- Dry skin

4. **How does estrogen affect the emotions of females?**

- Estrogen levels naturally fluctuate, but an imbalance can cause feelings of depression, anxiety, or mood changes. In some cases, doctors may prescribe estrogen therapy to help alleviate these effects.

Progesterone: The Hormonal Balance Restorer

Progesterone promotes menstruation and the early stages of pregnancy in women or people designated female at birth (AFAB). Progesterone deficiency might lead to pregnancy problems or menopausal symptoms.

Menstruation and progesterone

Ovulation (the release of an egg by the ovary) occurs in the middle of a woman's menstrual cycle. The corpus luteum develops from an empty egg follicle and begins to produce progesterone. If conception happens during that cycle, your corpus luteum is a transitory gland that assists in supporting the start of a pregnancy.

Progesterone works by thickening your uterine lining and promoting the implantation of a fertilized egg. If an egg is not fertilized during that cycle (you do not become pregnant), the corpus luteum breaks down, lowering progesterone levels. When your progesterone levels fall, your uterine lining thins and breaks down, resulting in the onset of your menstrual period.

Role of Progesterone in the Female Body:

Progesterone serves multiple functions, which encompass the following:

1. **Uterine Health:** Progesterone works in tandem with estrogen to regulate the menstrual cycle. It helps in regulating menstrual bleeding. It supports the development and thickness of the uterine lining and prepares it for potential embryo implantation.
2. **Pregnancy Support:** If pregnancy occurs, progesterone helps maintain the uterine lining and prevents contractions that could lead to miscarriage. It helps in sustaining a pregnancy after conception takes place.
3. **Breast Health:** Progesterone plays a role in breast development and health.
4. Assisting in mood enhancement.
5. Facilitating lactation.
6. Supporting the proper functioning of the thyroid.

Impact of Progesterone Decline in Menopause:

- **Menstrual Irregularities:** The decline in progesterone contributes to changes in the menstrual cycle, including irregular periods and eventual cessation.
- **Mood Swings:** Progesterone's influence on neurotransmitters can impact mood, potentially leading to mood swings and irritability.
- **Sleep Disturbances:** Changes in progesterone levels may contribute to sleep disturbances, affecting overall sleep quality.

The Unspoken Power of Testosterone

Testosterone is a vital hormone primarily synthesized by the gonads, which are the sex organs. In individuals assigned male at birth (AMAB), the testicles are responsible for testosterone production, while in individuals assigned female at birth (AFAB), it is the ovaries that produce this hormone. Additionally, the adrenal glands play a role in hormone production by producing dehydroepiandrosterone (DHEA), which can be converted into both testosterone and estrogen within the body.

As the primary androgen, testosterone plays a crucial role in promoting the development of male characteristics. It is worth noting that testosterone levels naturally tend to be significantly higher in individuals assigned male at birth (AMAB) compared to those assigned female at birth (AFAB).

Role of Testosterone in the Female Body:

Testosterone boosts libido in adults who were assigned female at birth. Nevertheless, the ovaries predominantly convert most of the testosterone they produce into estradiol, the primary female sex hormone.

Testosterone is a key factor in the development of sexual desire (libido) and plays a crucial role in arousal. It aids in the maintenance of muscle mass and strength, ensuring optimal physical performance. Testosterone has a direct impact on energy levels and overall vitality, promoting a sense of vigor and well-being. It exerts a positive influence on mood and cognitive function, contributing to emotional stability and mental clarity.

Impact of Testosterone Decline in Menopause:

- **Reduced Libido:** The decline in testosterone levels during menopause can result in a decrease in sexual desire, affecting overall sexual satisfaction.
- **Loss of Muscle Mass:** Fluctuations in testosterone levels can contribute to a gradual loss of muscle mass and strength, potentially impacting physical capabilities.

- **Fatigue and Mood Changes:** Lower testosterone levels experienced during menopause may be associated with changes in energy levels and mood, leading to feelings of fatigue and emotional instability.

Navigating the Transition: Understanding Hormonal Changes in Menopause

Menopause, a natural and transformative phase in a woman's life, is characterized by significant hormonal fluctuations that affect various aspects of physical and emotional well-being. Gaining an understanding of these hormonal changes is essential in order to comprehend the diverse symptoms associated with menopause and the role of Hormone Replacement Therapy (HRT) in restoring balance. Within this chapter, we delved into the intricate interplay of hormones during menopause and examined their impact on the female body.

The Importance of Hormonal Balance for Overall Well-being

Achieving and maintaining hormonal balance is a crucial part of the human body's complicated processes. Hormones thrive as messengers, regulating a complex set of physiological processes that affect one's physical well-being, emotional stability, and mental clarity. This section delves into the crucial role of hormonal balance in creating holistic well-being and analyzes how imbalances, particularly after menopause, may affect a woman's life in a variety of ways.

The state of hormonal balance is comparable to the body's equilibrium or homeostasis, where the levels of different hormones are finely tuned to meet the body's requirements. Optimal body functioning, including growth, metabolism, reproduction, and other vital processes, is supported when hormones are in balance. Hormones such as insulin and thyroid hormones play a critical role in metabolism, affecting energy levels and overall vitality.

Hormonal balance is also crucial for muscle health, strength, and endurance. Regular menstrual cycles and reproductive health are ensured by balanced levels of estrogen and progesterone. Hormonal balance is essential for fertility, influencing ovulation and overall reproductive capacity. Hormones like estrogen are also involved in calcium regulation, which is vital for maintaining strong and healthy bones. Hormonal balance supports bone density, reducing the risk of conditions like osteoporosis. Hormones also affect neurotransmitters like serotonin and dopamine, playing a role in mood regulation. Balanced cortisol levels contribute to a healthy stress response, preventing chronic stress-related issues.

Hormonal balance is linked to neurotransmitter harmony, reducing the risk of anxiety and depression. Exercise-induced endorphin release is influenced by hormonal balance, contributing to improved mood. Estrogen plays a role in cognitive function, influencing memory and concentration. Hormones contribute to neuroprotective effects, potentially reducing the risk of cognitive decline.

Chapter 3

The Evolution of Menopause Treatment Throughout History

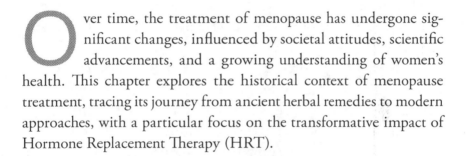

O ver time, the treatment of menopause has undergone significant changes, influenced by societal attitudes, scientific advancements, and a growing understanding of women's health. This chapter explores the historical context of menopause treatment, tracing its journey from ancient herbal remedies to modern approaches, with a particular focus on the transformative impact of Hormone Replacement Therapy (HRT).

Ancient Wisdom and Herbal Remedies

Across different cultures, menopause was often viewed through cultural lenses, with rituals and practices aimed at managing symptoms and maintaining health. Ancient societies relied on herbal remedies, with plants like black cohosh and soy gaining prominence for their perceived benefits in alleviating menopausal symptoms. The 19th century witnessed a shift towards medical explanations for menopause, moving away from solely cultural interpretations.

Early medical interventions included tonics and elixirs, often containing alcohol and various herbs, marketed to relieve menopausal discomfort. Menopause gained recognition as a medical condition rather than a cultural or psychological phenomenon. The mid-20th century saw the introduction of hormone therapies, initially using extracts from animal ovaries to alleviate menopausal symptoms.

The Pioneering Era of Hormone Replacement Therapy (HRT)

During the 1920s and 1930s, Serge Voronoff carried out a series of experiments where he transplanted slices of monkey testicles onto the testes of elderly men in an attempt to reverse the effects of aging. In parallel, researchers investigated the potential benefits of using extracts from animal glands, including ovaries and testes, as remedies for age-related symptoms. Through their studies, scientists were able to identify substances in ovarian tissues that possessed estrogenic properties. This discovery eventually led to the isolation of estrogenic compounds.

A significant milestone in the field came in 1938 with the synthesis of diethylstilbestrol (DES), which represented a major breakthrough. This synthetic estrogen offered a stable and potent form of estrogen, opening up new possibilities for medical applications.

In the 1940s, Wyeth Pharmaceuticals introduced Premarin, a conjugated estrogen product derived from pregnant mare's urine. It quickly became a widely prescribed hormone replacement therapy (HRT) for managing menopausal symptoms. However, concerns about the increased risk of uterine cancer with estrogen-only therapy prompted the introduction of progestins. Combining estrogen with a progestin became the standard practice, especially for women with a uterus.

The Women's Health Initiative, which began in 1991, was a large-scale clinical trial aimed at evaluating the long-term health benefits and risks of HRT. However, due to safety concerns, the study was terminated early in 2002. This raised questions about the risks associated with HRT and had an impact on its usage patterns. As an alternative to synthetic hormones, bioidentical hormones gained popularity. These hormones have a structure identical to those naturally produced in the body. Compounded bioidentical hormones allowed for personalized formulations tailored to individual needs.

The treatment of menopause has undergone significant changes over time, influenced by cultural beliefs, medical advancements, and shifting paradigms of women's health. From ancient remedies to controversial synthetic hormones, and now to a more personalized and integrative approach, the field of menopause treatment continues to evolve. Current trends in menopause care include a growing emphasis on holistic approaches. Complementary therapies, such as lifestyle modifications, nutrition, and mindfulness, are now considered as strategies to complement traditional treatments. Integrative medicine models have also emerged, blending conventional and complementary therapies to address menopause symptoms in a comprehensive manner.

Individualized Aspect of Modern Hormone Replacement Therapy (HRT)

In the realm of Hormone Replacement Therapy (HRT) today, there has been a significant shift towards providing personalized and individualized care. Recognizing that each woman's experience with menopause is unique, modern approaches to HRT prioritize tailoring treatment plans to meet specific needs, preferences, and health considerations. In this section, we will explore the key aspects that highlight the personalized nature of contemporary HRT:

1. **Thorough Assessment and Health History**

Holistic Understanding:

*   **Comprehensive Evaluation:** Modern HRT begins with a detailed assessment of a woman's health history, which includes medical conditions, family history, and lifestyle factors.

- **Analysis of Symptoms:** Understanding the nature and impact of menopausal symptoms provides crucial insights for creating personalized treatment plans.

2. **Customized Hormone Formulations**

Tailored Compounded Bioidentical Hormones:

- **Personalized Formulations:** Compounded bioidentical hormones allow for the customization of hormone formulations, aligning with an individual's specific hormonal needs.
- **Precision in Dosage:** The ability to precisely adjust the dosage and ratio of hormones contributes to a personalized and finely tuned approach.

3. **Targeted Management of Symptoms**

Addressing Specific Concerns:

- **Symptom-Focused Approach:** Contemporary HRT focuses on addressing specific menopausal symptoms that have the most significant impact on each woman.
- **Prioritizing Quality of Life:** Personalized treatment plans aim to enhance overall quality of life by alleviating symptoms that significantly affect well-being.

4. **Various Delivery Methods for Individual Preferences**

Flexible Administration Options:

- **Transdermal Patches, Oral Tablets, Sublingual Formulations:** The availability of diverse administration methods allows women to choose the option that aligns with their preferences and lifestyle.

- **Considering Individual Response:** Personalized care includes taking into account how an individual responds to different delivery methods and making adjustments accordingly.

5. Continuous Monitoring and Adaptations

Flexible Treatment Plans:

- **Regular Hormone Level Checks:** Consistent monitoring of hormone levels guarantees that treatment plans are in line with an individual's physiological response.
- **Adaptable Care:** The ability to make real-time adaptations based on ongoing assessments ensures that treatment remains optimized.

6. Holistic Approaches and Lifestyle Factors

Mind-Body Connection:

- **Comprehensive Integration:** Integrating complementary therapies, such as mindfulness, nutrition, and exercise, acknowledges the holistic nature of well-being.
- **Lifestyle Adjustments:** Personalized care emphasizes the integration of lifestyle adjustments, recognizing the impact of habits on overall health.

7. **Patient Education and Collaborative Decision-Making**

Empowering Women:

- **Informed Decision-Making:** Modern HRT prioritizes patient education, ensuring that women are well-informed about the potential benefits and risks.
- **Collaborative Decision-Making:** Shared decision-making between healthcare providers and patients empowers women to actively participate in determining their menopausal care.

8. **Long-Term Health Considerations**

Beyond Symptom Management:

- **Bone Health and Cardiovascular Considerations:** Personalized care extends beyond symptom relief to address long-term health considerations, such as bone health and cardiovascular health.
- **Cognitive Well-being:** Some contemporary approaches explore the potential benefits of HRT in maintaining cognitive function and reducing the risk of neurodegenerative conditions.

Chapter 4

Benefits and Risks of Hormone Replacement Therapy (HRT) on Menopausal Symptoms

I f you find yourself in the midst of experiencing menopause, rest assured that you are not alone. Every year, approximately 1.5 million women in the United States embark on the journey towards menopause, which is commonly referred to as perimenopause.

Perimenopause can commence as early as your 30s, triggered by natural biological changes that gradually decrease your hormone levels. Alternatively, it can occur suddenly due to the surgical removal of your uterus and ovaries, thrusting you into menopause almost instantaneously.

Menopause is a transformative phase, and Hormone Replacement Therapy (HRT) emerges as a valuable tool for women navigating the challenges associated with hormonal changes. In this section, we explore the positive impacts of HRT on various menopausal symptoms, empowering women to make informed decisions about their well-being.

Dr. Jessica Chan, a reproductive endocrinologist at Cedars-Sinai Fertility and Reproductive Medicine Center, explains that symptoms like brain fog, mood changes, hot flashes, and insomnia can leave you desperate for relief. Nowadays, hormone replacement therapy (HRT) is tailored to each woman's specific needs and potential risk factors. It is a collaborative decision-making process between the patient and their doctor.

According to Dr. Chan, there has been a shift in the attitude towards hormone therapy in recent years. Medical societies now advocate for not only using the lowest dose for the shortest duration but also using the appropriate dose for the appropriate amount of time. This personalized approach ensures that women receive the most effective and safe treatment for their symptoms.

HRT effectively alleviates menopausal symptoms by replenishing hormone levels. Additionally, it provides a safeguard against diseases like osteoporosis. The process of HRT typically involves the administration of estrogen and, if the uterus is intact, progestin (progesterone). Estrogen can be consumed in the form of pills, skin patches, or gels. In cases where progesterone is prescribed, it may be combined with estrogen in a pill or patch, although it is more commonly administered separately to prevent breakthrough bleeding.

Estrogen and progesterone are essential hormones in the human body. While progesterone primarily supports pregnancy and maintains the health of the uterus, estrogen serves various functions. Apart from its role in reproduction and the menstrual cycle, estrogen also safeguards bone health, reduces cholesterol levels, supports brain function through glucose metabolism, and maintains the vaginal lining.

According to Dr. Chan, estrogen is not limited to the reproductive system. It also has receptors in the brain, bones, heart, and blood vessels. Therefore, a decline in estrogen levels affects multiple systems in a woman's body. This is why menopausal women often experience cognitive decline, mood changes, and an increased risk of osteoporosis.

HRT Benefits & Risk

1. **Relieving Vasomotor Symptoms:** HRT has been found to effectively reduce the frequency and intensity of hot flashes, providing relief from this disruptive symptom. Additionally, by restoring hormonal balance, HRT can alleviate night sweats, promoting better sleep quality and overall comfort.

2. **Enhancing Vaginal Health:** Estrogen supplementation in HRT can address vaginal dryness, enhancing lubrication and reducing discomfort during intercourse. Furthermore, HRT supports the health of vaginal tissues, mitigating thinning that can lead to irritation and pain.

3. **Promoting Mood and Emotional Well-being:** HRT, particularly with the inclusion of progesterone, can help stabilize mood, reducing irritability and mood swings. Some studies also suggest that HRT may have positive effects on mood, potentially lowering the risk of depression and anxiety during menopause.

4. **Maintaining Bone Health:** Estrogen plays a crucial role in maintaining bone density, and HRT can contribute to reducing the risk of osteoporosis and fractures by supporting bone health. Women undergoing HRT will have a decreased risk of developing osteoporosis and those women who have osteopenia will see improved Z scores.

5. **Supporting Cognitive Function:** Estrogen has neuroprotective effects, and HRT may contribute to maintaining cognitive function, including memory and concentration. Additionally, some studies explore the potential benefits of HRT in reducing the risk of cognitive decline and neurodegenerative conditions.

6. **Improving Sexual Function:** Testosterone supplementation in HRT can enhance sexual desire, addressing concerns about decreased libido during menopause. HRT may also positively

impact orgasmic function, contributing to a more satisfying sexual experience.

7. **Improving Quality of Life:** Through the alleviation of troublesome symptoms, hormone replacement therapy (HRT) plays a significant role in enhancing the overall quality of life during the menopausal transition. By providing relief from symptoms, women are able to actively participate in their daily activities, promoting physical comfort and vitality.

Addressing Common Concerns and Dispelling Myths about Hormone Replacement Therapy (HRT)

As women contemplate Hormone Replacement Therapy (HRT) as a potential solution for alleviating menopausal symptoms, it is crucial to address common concerns and debunk prevailing misconceptions. Within this section, we aim to clarify misunderstandings surrounding HRT, empowering women to make well-informed decisions about their health:

1. **Breast Cancer Risk:**
   - **Concern:** One common misconception is that HRT substantially increases the risk of breast cancer.
   - **Reality:** The relationship between HRT and breast cancer is intricate. While certain studies suggest a slight increase in risk with long-term use, the overall risk is influenced by factors such as age, duration of use, and the specific hormones employed. Specifically, oral estrogen has been shown to cause an increased risk of breast cancer over the transdermal (gel or cream) from of estrogen.

2. **Cardiovascular Risks:**
   - **Concern:** There is a belief that HRT may heighten the risk of cardiovascular events, including heart attacks and strokes.

- **Reality:** Research indicates that the connection between HRT and cardiovascular health is multifaceted. In certain cases, particularly for younger women, HRT may offer cardiovascular benefits. However, individual risk factors should be taken into account.

3. **Blood Clot Risk:**
   - **Concern:** Some women worry about an elevated risk of blood clots associated with HRT usage.
   - **Reality:** Although HRT may have a slight association with blood clot risk, the overall risk is generally low. Individual risk factors, such as age, obesity, and smoking play a significant role.

4. **Weight Gain:**
   - **Concern:** There is a misconception that HRT leads to substantial weight gain.
   - **Reality:** Studies indicate that any weight gain associated with HRT is minimal and varies among individuals. Lifestyle factors, diet, and exercise have a more significant impact on weight during menopause.

5. **Natural and Bioidentical Hormones:**
   - **Concern:** Certain women hold the belief that natural or bioidentical hormones are inherently safer than synthetic hormones.
   - **Reality:** The safety of hormones, regardless of whether they are synthetic or bioidentical, relies on various factors. When prescribed and monitored correctly, both types of hormones can be safe and effective.

6. **Memory and Cognitive Concerns:**
   - **Concern:** There is a misconception that HRT has a negative impact on memory and cognitive function.

- **Reality:** Research indicates that HRT may potentially offer cognitive benefits, as some studies suggest a reduced risk of cognitive decline. However, individual responses to HRT can vary.

7. **HRT is Only for Severe Symptoms:**
   - **Concern:** Some women believe that HRT is exclusively suitable for severe menopausal symptoms.
   - **Reality:** HRT can provide benefits for a wide variety of symptoms, ranging from mild to severe. The decision to pursue HRT depends on individual symptoms, preferences, and overall health.

Personalized Risk-Benefit Analysis for Informed Decision-Making

When it comes to Hormone Replacement Therapy (HRT), the decision-making process is highly personalized. In this section, we will delve into the significance of conducting a personalized risk-benefit analysis. This analysis empowers women to make well-informed choices that are aligned with their unique health circumstances, preferences, and goals:

1. **Understanding the Individual's Health Profile:**
   a) **Health History:** A comprehensive evaluation of a woman's health history, which includes her family history, pre-existing conditions, and lifestyle factors, serves as the foundation for making personalized decisions.
   b) **Current Health Status:** Taking into account the individual's current health status, such as cardiovascular health, bone density, and cognitive function, provides valuable

insights into the potential benefits and risks associated with HRT.

2. **Identifying Menopausal Symptoms:**
   a) **Symptom Severity:** Assessing the severity of menopausal symptoms and their impact on daily life helps prioritize the need for symptom relief.
   b) **Specific Symptom Patterns:** Each woman may experience a unique combination of symptoms, and HRT can be tailored to address specific concerns.

3. **Establishing Personal Health Goals:**
   a) **Quality of Life:** Defining personal health goals in terms of overall well-being, quality of life, and maintaining a sense of vitality during menopause.
   b) **Long-Term Health Considerations:** Considering how HRT aligns with long-term health goals, including bone health, cardiovascular health, and cognitive well-being.

4. **Individualized Hormone Formulations:**
   a) **Bioidentical vs. Synthetic Hormones:** Exploring the choice between bioidentical and synthetic hormones, taking into account individual preferences and potential benefits. Bioidentical hormone replacement offers far less side effects compared to synthetic hormone replacement. This is crucial to speak to your provider about before starting hormone replacement therapy. Synthetic hormone replacement promotes side effects we commonly hear about associated with hormone replacement therapy.
   b) **Customized Formulations:** Considering the option of compounded bioidentical hormones to create personalized formulations based on specific hormonal needs.

5. **Risk Factors and Monitoring:**
   a) **Breast Cancer Risk Assessment:** Conducting an individualized assessment of breast cancer risk factors, considering factors such as age, family history, and lifestyle. Bioidentical hormone replacement therapy offers far less risk for breast cancer.
   b) **Cardiovascular Risk Evaluation:** Evaluating cardiovascular risk factors, including blood pressure, cholesterol levels, and overall heart health. Bioidentical hormone replacement therapy offers far less risk for cardiovascular accidents.
   c) **Blood Clot Risk Assessment:** Assessing individual risk factors for blood clots and considering alternatives or precautions as needed. Bioidentical hormone replacement therapy offers far less risk for blood clots.

6. **Addressing Emotional and Cognitive Well-being:**

When it comes to emotional health, it's important to consider the impact of menopausal symptoms and how hormone replacement therapy (HRT) can help stabilize mood. Additionally, cognitive health should be a priority, and HRT may also have potential benefits in maintaining cognitive function.

7. **Alternative Approaches and Lifestyle Modifications:**

In addition to HRT, it's worth exploring alternative approaches such as lifestyle modifications, nutrition, and complementary therapies. Engaging in shared decision-making with healthcare providers can also help ensure that the chosen approach is the best fit for your needs.

8. **Regular Monitoring and Adjustments:**

Menopause is a dynamic process, so it's important to implement treatment plans that can be adjusted based on frequent monitoring.

This responsive care approach ensures that your chosen approach remains aligned with your evolving health needs and goals.

The initiation of Hormone Replacement Therapy (HRT) marks the commencement of a dynamic journey, and the significance of continuous monitoring and modifications cannot be emphasized enough. In this segment, we explore into the reasons why ongoing evaluation and adjustments to the treatment plan are essential for optimizing outcomes and ensuring the well-being of women during the menopausal phase.

Menopause is characterized by fluctuating hormone levels, which makes each woman's experience unique. Menopausal symptoms may change over time, necessitating modifications to the treatment plan. Women respond differently to HRT based on factors such as genetics, lifestyle, and overall health. Continuous monitoring enables the customization of treatment plans to address individual responses and requirements.

Menopausal symptoms are often subjective and can vary in intensity. Regular monitoring enables healthcare providers to evaluate the degree of symptom relief and make adjustments as necessary. Periodic checks of hormone levels help ensure that they remain within the desired therapeutic range. Modifying hormone dosages based on laboratory results helps maintain balance and optimize treatment outcomes.

Continuous monitoring enables the timely identification of any potential side effects or adverse reactions. If side effects occur, adjustments to the type or dosage of hormones may be necessary to minimize discomfort. Regular assessments of bone density help evaluate the impact of HRT on long-term bone health.

Monitoring cardiovascular health indicators ensures that the chosen treatment aligns with long-term cardiovascular well-being. As women progress through menopause, their health goals may change. Continuous monitoring allows for the reassessment and adjustment of treatment plans to align with changing health priorities. Establishing open communication between women and their healthcare providers is crucial. Regular check-ins facilitate shared decision-making, where women actively participate in their care.

Chapter 5

Integrating Lifestyle Modifications with Hormone Replacement Therapy

The integration of lifestyle modifications with hormone replacement therapy (HRT) is a comprehensive approach aimed at optimizing overall health and well-being. HRT is commonly used to address hormonal imbalances that may arise due to aging, medical conditions, or other factors. However, the effectiveness of HRT can be further enhanced when combined with lifestyle modifications.

To begin, dietary choices play a critical role in hormone balance. A diet rich in nutrient-dense foods, such as fruits, vegetables, and whole grains, provides essential vitamins and minerals crucial for hormonal production and regulation. Additionally, incorporating sufficient protein and healthy fats supports hormonal synthesis. Tailoring the diet to specific hormonal needs, such as ensuring an adequate intake of omega-3 fatty acids for optimal brain function or incorporating foods with phytoestrogens for women undergoing estrogen replacement, can complement HRT.

Regular physical activity is another essential component of this integrated approach. Exercise not only aids in weight management, which is crucial for hormonal balance, but also stimulates the production of endorphins, contributing to improved mood and overall well-being. Furthermore, resistance training has been shown to positively impact bone density, an important consideration in the context of hormonal changes, especially in postmenopausal women.

Adequate sleep is often overlooked but is critical for hormone regulation and overall health. Hormones such as growth hormone and cortisol follow a circadian rhythm, and disruptions in sleep patterns can lead to imbalances. Integrating strategies to improve sleep hygiene, such as maintaining a consistent sleep schedule and creating a conducive sleep environment, can complement the benefits of HRT.

Stress management methods also have a vital role in enhancing hormonal well-being. Prolonged stress can result in increased cortisol levels, which can negatively impact other hormonal processes. Techniques like meditation, mindfulness, and relaxation exercises can be incorporated to alleviate stress and bolster the beneficial outcomes of hormone replacement therapy.

The Synergy of Lifestyle and Hormonal Balance

The interplay between lifestyle choices and hormonal balance is a dynamic process that significantly impacts overall health and well-being. Hormones act as messengers in the body, regulating essential processes such as metabolism, mood, and reproductive functions. Lifestyle factors, including diet, exercise, sleep, and stress management, intricately interact with hormonal systems, creating a delicate balance.

Nutrition plays a crucial role in hormonal balance, as the nutrients derived from food act as building blocks for hormone synthesis. A well-balanced diet, rich in vitamins, minerals, and macronutrients, supports optimal hormonal production. For example, incorporating omega-3 fatty acids can positively impact brain health and mood, while a diet with adequate protein contributes to muscle development and hormone synthesis.

Regular physical activity is another key factor in maintaining hormonal equilibrium. Exercise not only aids in weight management but also stimulates the release of endorphins, promoting a positive mood and reducing stress. Additionally, specific types of exercise, such as strength training, can influence hormones like insulin and growth hormone, contributing to metabolic health and muscle maintenance.

The significance of sleep in hormonal regulation cannot be overstated. During sleep, the body undergoes crucial processes of repair and regeneration, including the release of growth hormone. Disruptions in sleep patterns can lead to imbalances in hormones like cortisol and insulin, impacting metabolism and stress response. Prioritizing sufficient and quality sleep is thus integral to supporting hormonal harmony.

Stress management strategies are crucial in maintaining a harmonious hormonal balance and overall well-being. Prolonged stress can result in excessive cortisol production, which disrupts the equilibrium of other hormones and gives rise to a range of health problems. By embracing mindfulness techniques, engaging in meditation, or practicing relaxation exercises, one can effectively counteract the adverse impact of stress and cultivate a more balanced hormonal environment.

Nutrition as a Foundation:

Nutrition plays a vital role in promoting overall health and well-being, serving as the foundation for optimal physiological processes and vital bodily functions. The popular saying "you are what you eat" emphasizes the significant impact of dietary choices on individual health. It is crucial to maintain a well-balanced and nutrient-rich diet to provide the body with the necessary components for growth, energy production, and maintenance.

Macronutrients, which include carbohydrates, proteins, and fats, are essential elements of a healthy diet. Carbohydrates serve as the primary source of energy, proteins contribute to tissue repair and synthesis, and fats are crucial for cell structure and hormone production. Striking the right balance among these macronutrients ensures a consistent and sustainable supply of energy while supporting various physiological functions. Equally important are micronutrients, such as vitamins and minerals, in maintaining good health. These micronutrients act as co-factors in enzymatic reactions, facilitating processes like metabolism and immune function. For instance, vitamin C plays a critical role in collagen synthesis and immune system support, while minerals like calcium and phosphorus are necessary for maintaining strong bones.

The quality of food choices is just as significant as the quantity. Opting for whole, unprocessed foods like fruits, vegetables, whole grains, lean proteins, and healthy fats provides a diverse range of nutrients with optimal bioavailability. On the other hand, a diet high in processed foods, refined sugars, and excessive saturated fats can lead to nutritional deficiencies and health problems.

Nutrition has a profound impact on both physical health and mental well-being. It is not only essential for maintaining a healthy body but also plays a crucial role in cognitive function and mood regulation. Omega-3 fatty acids, which are abundant in fish, have been associated with improved cognitive abilities and the regulation of mood. Furthermore, a well-balanced diet that helps maintain stable blood sugar levels can greatly influence concentration, mood stability, and overall mental clarity. The significance of nutrition goes beyond individual well-being and extends to the overall health of society. It is imperative to address the issue of malnutrition, including both undernutrition and overnutrition, in order to promote public health and prevent the onset of various chronic diseases.

Exercise for Physical Vitality:

Regular physical exercise is essential for achieving and maintaining physical well-being. It goes beyond just helping with weight management and offers numerous benefits for cardiovascular health, muscular strength, and mental resilience. Exercise is not simply a fitness routine; it is a comprehensive approach to rejuvenating the body and optimizing its functions.

Cardiovascular exercises like brisk walking, running, or cycling are crucial for improving heart health. These activities increase the heart rate, ensuring efficient blood circulation and oxygen delivery to tissues and organs. Over time, cardiovascular exercise strengthens the heart, lowers blood pressure, and reduces the risk of cardiovascular diseases, promoting vitality and longevity.

Strength training, which includes weightlifting and bodyweight exercises, plays a vital role in building and preserving muscle mass. In addition to sculpting a toned physique, strong muscles contribute to better posture, joint stability, and overall functional fitness. This is particularly important for supporting daily activities and preventing injuries, enabling individuals to maintain an active and vibrant lifestyle.

Flexibility and balance exercises, such as yoga or tai chi, are essential for enhancing overall physical function. These activities improve joint range of motion, flexibility, and balance, reducing the risk of falls and injuries, especially in older adults. Incorporating these exercises into a fitness routine ensures a well-rounded approach to physical vitality.

Regular exercise not only benefits physical health but also has a positive impact on mental and emotional well-being. The release of endorphins during physical activity contributes to improved mood and stress reduction, making exercise a powerful antidote to the challenges of daily life. To fully unlock the potential of exercise for physical vitality, consistency is key. Establishing a regular routine that includes a variety of cardiovascular, strength, and flexibility exercises ensures a comprehensive approach to fitness. Tailoring the exercise regimen to individual preferences and fitness levels enhances adherence, making it more likely to become a sustainable and enjoyable part of daily life.

Mindfulness and Stress Management:

In today's fast-paced world, stress has become a common problem for many individuals. However, mindfulness can serve as a powerful tool for stress management. By cultivating awareness and being present in the current moment without judgment, individuals can shift their perception and response to stressors. Mindfulness involves paying attention to one's thoughts, emotions, and physical sensations with a non-judgmental attitude, allowing individuals to observe stressors without becoming overwhelmed by them.

Techniques such as meditation, deep breathing, and body scans can anchor individuals in the present moment and alleviate the impact of stress. One of the key benefits of mindfulness is its ability to break the cycle of automatic reactions, allowing for a more measured and intentional response to stress. Regular practice of mindfulness can also physiologically impact the body's stress response, promoting overall relaxation and resilience to chronic stress.

Mindfulness not only has an immediate calming effect, but it also promotes resilience in the face of stress. By accepting the present moment and acknowledging challenges without judgment, individuals can develop a more adaptive and positive outlook. This shift in perspective not only mitigates the impact of stress but also cultivates emotional well-being and mental clarity. Incorporating mindfulness into daily life is a gradual process that often begins with short, regular sessions. These sessions can be as simple as focusing on the breath, observing thoughts without attachment, or practicing mindful walking.

Over time, individuals can integrate mindfulness into various aspects of their routine, making it a natural and sustainable part of their approach to stress management.

Complementary Therapies:

Complementary therapies, also known as alternative or integrative therapies, encompass a wide range of approaches that are used alongside conventional medical treatments to enhance overall well-being and address various health conditions. These therapies acknowledge the interconnection between the mind, body, and spirit, with the goal of supporting the body's natural healing processes and augmenting the effectiveness of traditional medical interventions.

One commonly embraced complementary therapy is acupuncture, which originates from traditional Chinese medicine. This practice involves the insertion of thin needles into specific points on the body to stimulate the flow of energy, known as Qi, and promote equilibrium. Acupuncture has been utilized to alleviate pain, manage stress, and address a variety of health issues, and its integration with mainstream medicine is increasingly acknowledged for its potential benefits.

Another popular complementary therapy is massage therapy, which entails the manipulation of soft tissues to induce relaxation, reduce muscle tension, and enhance circulation. Beyond its physical advantages, massage therapy is frequently employed to alleviate stress, anxiety, and promote mental well-being. Many healthcare professionals incorporate massage as part of rehabilitation or pain management programs.

Mind-body practices, such as yoga and meditation, are integral components of complementary therapies. These techniques emphasize the connection between mental and physical health, fostering relaxation, stress reduction, and improved mental clarity. For example, yoga combines physical postures, breath control, and meditation to enhance flexibility, balance, and overall well-being.

The practice of herbal medicine, also known as botanical medicine, involves the use of plant-based remedies to address a variety of health concerns. Herbal supplements, teas, and tinctures are frequently utilized to support the body's natural healing processes. Although the effectiveness of herbal remedies can vary, certain herbs have been shown to possess therapeutic properties and are used in conjunction with traditional treatments.

Chiropractic care is another form of complementary therapy that concentrates on the musculoskeletal system, particularly the spine. Chiropractors employ manual adjustments to correct misalignments, with the goal of enhancing nerve function and overall health. This method is frequently employed to manage conditions such as back pain and headaches.

It is important to note that the integration of complementary therapies into healthcare is frequently based on an individual's preferences, the nature of their health condition, and collaboration with healthcare professionals. To ensure that complementary therapies align with overall treatment goals and do not interfere with conventional medical interventions, open communication between patients and healthcare providers is critical.

Maintaining a Healthy Weight:

Ensuring a healthy weight is crucial for overall well-being, as it helps prevent various health conditions and promotes an active lifestyle. To achieve and maintain a healthy weight, it is important to adopt a balanced diet, engage in regular physical activity, and make mindful lifestyle choices. The role of diet in weight management cannot be overstated. A nutrient-dense diet that includes a variety of fruits, vegetables, whole grains, lean proteins, and healthy fats is essential for providing the body with necessary nutrients while promoting a feeling of fullness.

Portion control is also important to regulate caloric intake and prevent overeating. Staying hydrated is equally important, as thirst can sometimes be mistaken for hunger. Balancing macronutrients, such as carbohydrates, proteins, and fats, is crucial for sustained energy levels and regulating metabolic processes. Incorporating fiber-rich foods aids in digestion and reduces the likelihood of overindulging in less nutritious options. Minimizing the intake of processed foods, sugary beverages, and excessive amounts of saturated fats is also important for overall health and weight management.

Regular physical activity is another key component of maintaining a healthy weight. A combination of aerobic exercises, such as walking, running, or cycling, and strength training activities helps burn calories, build muscle, and boost metabolism. Finding enjoyable forms of exercise increases the likelihood of long-term adherence to a fitness routine, making physical activity a sustainable and rewarding habit.

Sleep is often overlooked in discussions about weight management, but it plays a significant role. Sleep deprivation can disrupt hormonal balance, leading to increased feelings of hunger and a tendency to choose less healthy food options. Prioritizing quality sleep supports overall health and contributes to weight maintenance.

Mindful eating practices also play a vital role in weight management. Paying attention to hunger and fullness cues, savoring each bite, and avoiding distractions during meals can promote a healthier relationship with food. Emotional eating, often triggered by stress or other emotions, can be addressed through alternative coping mechanisms, such as engaging in hobbies or seeking support from friends and family.

Effective weight management involves a comprehensive approach that goes beyond just physical aspects and includes mental and emotional well-being. Developing a positive body image and adopting a realistic mindset towards weight goals are crucial for a sustainable and balanced approach. Instead of fixating on numbers on a scale, it is important to focus on overall health to gain a more holistic understanding of well-being.

Limiting Alcohol and Tobacco Use:

Prioritizing cardiovascular health requires conscious decision-making, and two important factors to take into account are reducing alcohol consumption and avoiding tobacco use. These lifestyle choices are particularly significant when considering the cardiovascular effects of Hormone Replacement Therapy (HRT).

To begin with, it is crucial to limit alcohol intake in order to maintain a healthy cardiovascular system. While moderate alcohol consumption may have some cardiovascular benefits, excessive or chronic alcohol consumption can contribute to high blood pressure, irregular heartbeats, and cardiomyopathy. These conditions can worsen the cardiovascular effects of hormone replacement therapy. Therefore, it is advisable to adhere to recommended alcohol limits, which typically suggest moderate consumption for both men and women.

Avoiding tobacco use is of utmost importance for cardiovascular health, especially in the context of HRT. Smoking is a well-known risk factor for heart disease, and when combined with the hormonal changes introduced through HRT, the potential for cardiovascular complications may increase. Tobacco use not only accelerates the progression of atherosclerosis but also poses additional risks for blood clots, which can further compound the cardiovascular impact of hormonal therapies. Hence, maintaining a smoke-free lifestyle is essential for individuals undergoing or considering hormone replacement therapy.

In addition to these specific considerations, promoting overall health by minimizing lifestyle factors that contribute to disease risk is crucial. Taking a holistic approach involves maintaining a balanced diet, engaging in regular physical activity, managing stress, and ensuring adequate sleep. These lifestyle factors work together synergistically to promote cardiovascular health and can enhance the positive effects of HRT.

A heart-healthy diet that includes plenty of fruits, vegetables, whole grains, lean proteins, and healthy fats supports cardiovascular well-being. Regular physical activity helps manage weight, lower blood pressure, and improve cholesterol levels.

Conclusion

This guide empowers women with knowledge on menopause and Hormone Replacement Therapy (HRT). Menopause, a natural process in the late 40s to early 50s, brings symptoms like hot flashes and mood swings. HRT, supplementing hormones, aims to alleviate symptoms and restore balance.

Key points include personalized treatment plans, lifestyle integration for holistic care, and ongoing monitoring. Success stories illustrate the transformative power of HRT and lifestyle changes. Looking ahead, advancements in research may refine treatments, holistic care models will prioritize individualized plans, patient-centered solutions will empower women, and technological integration may enhance accessibility and monitoring in menopause care. The purpose of this book is to educate the female patient on the importance of seeking out hormone replacement therapy when their menopause symptoms start. In today's word, the onset of menopause is getting younger and younger. It is vital to seek treatment early in order to minimize the symptoms associated menopause. Treatment should be sought after by a hormone specialist who specializes in hormone replacement and is familiar in bioidentical hormone replacement.

—Derek Lambert, NP

References

1   Northrup, C. M. (2012). *The Wisdom of Menopause: Creating Physical and Emotional Health During the Change*. Bantam.

2   Eyre, R. S. (2017). *Feeling Fat, Fuzzy, or Frazzled?: A 3-Step Program to: Restore Thyroid, Adrenal, and Reproductive Balance, Beat Hormone Havoc, and Feel Better Fast! Grand Central Life & Style*.

3   Prior, J. C. (2006). *Estrogen's Storm Season: Stories of Perimenopause*. Centre for Menstrual Cycle and Ovulation Research.

4   Machelle M. S. (2018). *The Menopause Diet: A Natural Guide to Managing Hormones, Health, and Happiness*. Robert Rose.

5   Gottfried, S. (2019). *Brain Body Diet: 40 Days to a Lean, Calm, Energized, and Happy Self*. HarperOne.

6   Bachmann, G. A. (2018). *The Menopause Answer Book: Practical Answers, Treatments, and Solutions for Your Unique Symptoms*. Sourcebooks.

7   Roizen, M. F., & Oz, M. C. (2014). *You: Staying Young: The Owner's Manual for Extending Your Warranty*. Free Press.

8   Nelson, H. D. (2012). *Menopause Practice: A Clinician's Guide*. Humana Press.

9   Kraemer, G. R. (2019). *Hormones and Your Health: The Smart Woman's Guide to Hormonal and Alternative Therapies for Menopause*. McFarland.

10 Richmond, V. L. (2007). *Taking Charge of Your Own Health: Navigating Your Way Through Diagnosis, Treatment, Insurance, and More*. Capital Books.

Printed in the United States
by Baker & Taylor Publisher Services